Foreword

The purpose of The Integrated Care Pathways Guide to Good Practice is to assist clinical teams with the implementation of Integrated Care Pathways (ICPs) in Wales. This Guide is the legacy of the ICP Network that was supported by Innovations in Care at the Welsh Assembly Government from June 2003 to October 2004. The Network was widely attended by representatives from across all NHS Trusts, Local Health Boards and the wider health community. This Guide is intended to ensure that there is equity in the development of ICPs across Wales and gives the reader helpful suggestions to develop and establish successful and sustainable ICPs.

Designed for Life[1] has set the NHS some challenging targets for the next ten years as we work to create world class health care and social services for Wales. The development of Integrated Care Pathways will be central to achieving those targets.

Acknowledgements

We would like to thank Allan Cumming (Associate Director for Service Development, National Leadership and Innovation Agency for Healthcare) for his support to the Network and the publication of this guide. We also thank the Network for their assistance in producing this ICP Good Practice Guide and Jayne Gibbs for all the administrative support given.

The Authoring Team

- Nicola Davis, ICP Development Manager, Swansea Local Health Board (formerly ICP Programme Lead, Innovations in Care)

- Grace Sansom, ICP Development Manager, Swansea NHS Trust

- Sian Jones, ICP Manager, Cardiff and Vale NHS Trust

- Kellie Jenkins, Deputy Clinical Governance Manager, Pontypridd and Rhondda NHS Trust

- Lucy Roberts, ICP Co-ordinator, North East Wales NHS Trust and Wrexham and Flintshire Local Health Boards

- Debbie Doig-Evans, ICP Facilitator, Conwy and Denbighshire NHS Trust.

- Nia Richards, Sevice Development Manager, NLIAH

1 Designed for Life: Creating World Class Health and Social Care for Wales in the 21st Century; Welsh Assembly Government, 2005

Contents

Chapter 1:   **The Integrated Care Pathway**   5
   1.1   What is an Integrated Care Pathway   7
   1.2   All Wales Integrated Care Pathway Network Standards   8
   1.3   Modernisation in the UK and USA   11
   1.4   Culture and the Human Dimensions of Change   13

Chapter 2:   **Developing an Integrated Care Pathway**   15
   2.1   Developing your Integrated Care Pathway   22
   2.2   The Four Meeting Model   30

Chapter 3:   **Variances and Variance Tracking**   36

Chapter 4:   **Continuous Review and Improvement**   38
   4.1   The Future of ICPs   39
   4.2   The Birmingham Integrated Care Pathway Appraisal Tool   40

Appendix 1   Putting Patients at the Centre of Care   43
Appendix 2   Recommendations for Design and Layout   45
Appendix 3   ICP Timeline   48
Appendix 4   The Venture Good Integrated Care Pathway Template Matrix   50
Appendix 5   Impact Plan and Evaluation   53
Appendix 6   Glossary   54
Appendix 7   Useful Resources   56

The Integrated Care Pathway

ICPs come under the umbrella of a set of tools known as 'structured care methodologies'; tools that formalise known patterns of care processes, thus adding predictability and providing the transfer of knowledge.

Research protocols, guidelines, algorithms and the problem orientated medical record are all examples of structured care methodologies.

History of Developments

1985 – 1986	Invented at New England Medical Centre, Boston; begun as case managements plans then critical paths and evolved to care map® medical record
	First Wave
1986 – 1988	US 'early adopters' were hospitals in the States with high Medicare patient volume; Arizona, Florida, Rhode Island. For high Volume surgical populations such as orthopaedics, coronary artery bypass grafts.
1989 +	Applications in Australia and UK
	Second Wave
Mid – 1990	Spain (Catalonia), New Zealand, South Africa and Saudi Arabia.
	Third Wave
	Belgium, Japan, Singapore, Germany
	Fourth Wave
	Korea, Ecuador

There have been numerous government documents and Welsh Assembly Government revised documents which mention ICPs and patient journeys.

■ Putting Patients First (1998)

■ Quality Care Clinical Excellence (1999)

■ Improving Health in Wales: A plan for the NHS with its Partners (Feb 2001)

■ Wanless - Review of Health and Social Care in Wales (2004)

■ Designed for Life: Creating World Class Health and Social Care for Wales in the 21st Century (2005)

Emerging National Service Frameworks (NSFs) and National Institute of Clinical Excellence (NICE) guidelines all support the developments of ICPs.

The National Leadership and Innovation Agency for Healthcare in Wales (NLIAH) and the Clinical Support and Development Unit at the Welsh Assembly Government are keen to support ICP development in Wales.

The ICP network ran from June 2003 until October 2004. The main aim of the programme was to influence the concept of ICPs as a way for Clinicians to deliver clinically effective care to support the Clinical Governance agenda. Visits to the Chief Executives, Medical and Nurse Directors of Trusts and Local Health Boards around Wales to promote ICP concepts were received positively.

The initial Network meeting was formal and the audience widespread with speakers such as Professor P Degeling and Dr B Ferguson, who have undertaken research on the benefits of ICPs within Wales, Northern England and Australia. The subsequent Network meetings saw the numbers of participating health communities rise and the number of ICP managers appointed in Wales increase until it became the way forward within the 'governance and modernisation teams' in each health community. The experience within the Network for advice and experience on ICP development was second to none.

What is an Integrated Care Pathway?

An ICP is a document that describes a process within Health and Social Care. ICPs are both a tool and a concept which embed guidelines, protocols and locally agreed, evidence-based, patient-centred, best practice into everyday use for the individual patient. Uniquely to ICPs they record variations from planned care in the form of 'variances'.

An ICP aims to have:
- The right people ■ In the right order ■ In the right place
- Doing the right thing ■ In the right time ■ With the right outcomes
- All with attention to the patient experience

Appendix 1 contains a diagram which explains how patients are put at the centre of care.

The ICP is structured around the 'variance tracking tool' (real time audit) and it describes a process for a discreet element of care, for example, primary care, admission, acute care, rehabilitation or discharge. These elements build together to construct a unique journey for each individual patient according to their needs, based on professional judgement. For example, a diabetic journey may include a Deep Vein Thrombosis (DVT) element where necessary.
It sets out anticipated, evidence-based, best practice and outcomes that are locally agreed and that reflect a patient-centred, multi-disciplinary, multi-agency approach. It must be noted that although certain elements of care can be entirely 'unidisciplinary', they cannot be constructed without the knowledge and input of the whole multidisciplinary team.

The ICP document becomes all or part of the contemporaneous patient/client record. Completed activities, outcomes and variations between planned and actual care are recorded at the point of delivery.

There is much evidence showing that ICPs have a positive affect on particular patient conditions. Further UK research is needed to provide evidence that ICPs make a difference in generic terms. There is work as yet unpublished in the English language from the Belgian–Dutch Clinical ICP Network which shows evidence that ICPs do make a difference.

Even if the evidence to support the fact that ICPs do make a difference is currently limited, it is apparent that ICPs show their worth in enabling the smooth implementation of current guidelines such as NSFs, NICE Guidelines and health communities' individual clinical governance guidelines. ICPs can certainly demonstrate their value by offering a continual, real time audit via variance tracking which can contribute to all quality and effectiveness agendas.

"The development and implementation of ICPs is an integral part of both Quality and Modernisation agendas across Health Communities. ICPs are key to reducing the variation in healthcare, which can lead to cost savings and lower waiting times. ICPs are crucial to ensuring the delivery of care that is safe, effective, patient centred, timely, efficient and equitable in the NHS."

Nicola Davis - Integrated Care Pathway Network 2004

The term 'Integrated Care Pathway' is often misused and there are many so called 'ICPs' being developed and implemented across Wales with no uniformity. One objective of the Innovations in Care ICP Programme was to develop the standards for the elements that make up an ICP. These were drawn up not for performance management purposes but to enable a measurement guide to assist in the development of ICPs.

The Gold Standard for development for ICPs as agreed by the ICP Network 2003

An ICP is anticipated care placed in an appropriate time frame, written and agreed by a multidisciplinary team. It has locally agreed standards based on evidence where available to help a patient with a specific condition or diagnosis move progressively through the clinical experience. It forms part or all of the clinical record, documenting the care given. It facilitates and demonstrates continuous quality improvement. It includes patient milestones and clinical interventions noted on the day or stage that they are expected to occur. It will include all of the following standards or show evidence that it is working towards meeting these standards:

- Multidisciplinary
- Single Documentation
- Use exception reporting
- Variance analysis
- Patient/user involvement
- Monitoring of the utilisation

- Cross Boundaries
- Standard Format
- Outcome orientated
- Built in audit
- Evidence based

Innovations in Care, Welsh Assembly Government 2003

Common questions

Why must ICPs be Multidisciplinary?

ICPs should be developed by a multidisciplinary team and should deal with all aspects of patient care. Existing individual speciality or professionally based ICPs (e.g. nursing, medical and allied health professional notes) should be incorporated into the ICP document. This is essential to ensure patient focused care, supporting the streamlining of services, improved communication, and improved patient outcomes.

Why is it important to work across professional/organisational boundaries?

Since the patient journey crosses organisational boundaries both internal and external, ICPs should reflect this process.

What happens to existing documentation?

ICP documentation should include all documentation associated with the patient's care. Separate documents for different professional groups and organisations need to be incorporated into the ICP so that all information relevant to the patient is available to all members of the team wherever possible.

Why use a standard format?

A standard format for ICP documentation within an organisation will mean that staff dealing with multiple ICPs will find it easier to locate key information, as discreet elements should bolt together. The idea of a common 'look and feel' in documentation will also help in raising the profile of ICPs in organisations and reduce resistance and improve implementation.

What is exception reporting?

Wherever possible, reporting on ICPs should be by exception, within agreed standards. Entries in to the ICP should either be initialled to confirm that the expected standard is met or details should be given as to why or where the standard has not been met.

What is outcome orientated care?

ICPs should focus on outcomes. Standards should be set for patients as they progress through their care journey and achieve key milestones. This allows variations in care to be correlated with exceptions in outcomes to determine how care or the ICP itself could be improved.

Why clinical judgement is of the utmost importance?

ICPs are intended as a guide to providing care for patients and their families. Professionals are encouraged to exercise their own judgement, however, any alteration to the practice identified within the ICP must be recorded as a variance. If appropriate, patients can stop using the ICP 'care package' at any time, if clinical judgement deems it appropriate.

What is variance tracking and analysis?

All ICPs should have a mechanism to undertake regular analysis of variations. Variance analysis where outcomes are recorded gives a mechanism for determining the impact of variation in care and allows the ICP to be used as a tool for supporting clinical governance and audit. Variance analysis also allows changes to the ICP to be evaluated, making the ICP a living document.

How do ICPs fit with clinical governance?

ICPs are interlinked to all aspects of clinical governance. ICPs are related to the clinical governance initiative to implement standardised, best-practice clinical management in healthcare organisations. A regular multidisciplinary review of variances allows all clinical staff to have input into clinical audit. All ICPs should consider risks relevant to the specific condition and where appropriate develop the ICP in such a way so as to reduce patient risks.

ICPs can be used to help to continuously monitor and improve clinical quality by:

- including explicit clinical standards

- providing a system for clinical record keeping

- incorporating evidence-based guidelines for everyday practice

- identifying and managing risk

Can you have patient involvement in ICP development?

Yes, ICP development should involve patients where appropriate by the use of tools mentioned later in the guide. Patient representatives can also be involved, within the bounds of confidentiality, in ICP development and variance analysis

Ultimately it should may be the aim of the specific ICP development teams within Trusts and LHBs to develop a patient version of the ICP.

What if there is no evidence base?

ICPs should be based on evidence where evidence is available. Whilst it may take some time to reach the standard that all ICPs are evidence based, this should be the goal. However, lack of agreement on evidence based standards for a condition, or lack of national standards, should not be seen as a barrier to ICP development. As a first step, internally consistent custom and best practice should be adopted as the ICP standard.

The Unified Assessment and Care Management system (UACM) was developed in 2002, by the Social Services Inspectorate for Wales (SSIW).

The purpose of UACM is to ensure that agencies take a holistic approach to assessing and managing care and work together so that;-

- Assessment and care planning is person-centred and proportionate to need.

- Services are co-ordinated and integrated at all levels.

- Duplication of information, assessments and paperwork is minimised with advantages for individuals, practitioners and services.

- Eligibility criteria are fairer and standardised.

The UACM message is comparable to the principles of ICPs.

Modernisation in the UK and USA

The NHS Plan 'Improving Health in Wales' set out a vision for the future development of the NHS in Wales where every part is forward thinking, innovative and modern; 'a renewed NHS'. It is recognised that to modernise, investment in services needs to be combined with a fresh look at how we do things in order to start to do things differently.

A key driver for the establishment of the NLIAH was the Review of Health and Social Care in Wales (Wanless, 2002), which identified that healthcare in Wales would no longer be sustainable unless significant efforts were made to bring about real improvements. The Wanless interim report specified what patients and the public will expect of the NHS :

- safe, high quality treatment

- fast access

- an integrated, joined-up system

- comfortable accommodation services

- a patient-centred service.

Innovations in Care, the predecessor to NLIAH, was introduced by the Welsh Assembly Government in 2000 with four main aims:

- Recognising and spreading good practice

- Delivering improvement programmes

- Creating an improvement culture

- Advising on healthcare policy

The sister organisation in England, the Modernisation Agency was established in April 2001 (and it's successor, The Institute for Learning, Skills and Innovation, formed in July 2005). The NLIAH has also focused on four areas:

- improving access

- increasing local support

- raising standards of care

- capturing and sharing knowledge widely

ICP developments will play a key part in both service redesign and monitoring of best practice as the NLIAH works to help the health and social care community deliver Vision 2005.

In 'Designed for Life' a new vision is set out for health and social care in Wales[1].

The Institute for Healthcare Improvement (IHI)[2] is an American organisation committed to improving healthcare for people all over the world. The following six headings; safety, effectiveness, patient centredness, timeliness, efficiency and equity are central to IHI's focus on service redesign. Examples of how ICPs relate to each heading are discussed below:

- **Safety:** Healthcare is not safe, in absolute terms or in comparison to other industries or activities. The NHS must continually strive to make healthcare safer for patients. Trusts should work closely with the National Patient Safety Agency and implement ICPs where they can help reduce unsafe practices, by giving clinical teams the most up to date evidence on which to base care.

- **Effectiveness:** The NHS must continually work to improve the effectiveness of clinical services. Administrative processes and procedures must ensure that the patient receives care from the right professional in the right way and in the right location. Where there is evidence that a procedure or treatment is effective, that treatment must be offered to those that need it. Where there is no evidence that a procedure or treatment is effective, it should not be offered.

- **Patient Centredness:** All care should be centred around the patient's experience. ICPs are the perfect tool to involve patients in their own care. In some areas 'patient ICPs' have been developed in conjunction with 'clinical ICPs'. This is an effective education and information tool for patients and also demonstrates that communication channels are becoming more and more transparent.

- **Timeliness:** Care should be delivered in a timely way. ICPs reduce variation in the delivery of care and consequently reduce waiting times. This will ensure that patients are seen by the appropriate health professional according to their clinical need.

- **Efficiency:** All money wasted in the NHS is money that could be spent on patient care. ICPs can improve efficiency by avoiding duplication, streamlining care, reducing inefficient practices and keeping waste to a minimum.

- **Equity:** ICPs can standardise care, where appropriate, ensuring that it is patient focused outcomes that are measured and bias such as the 'postcode lottery' is eradicated.

1 *Designed for Life: Creating World Class Health and Social Care for Wales in the 21st Century;* Welsh Assembly Government, 2005

2 *www.ihi.org*

Culture and the Human Dimension of Change

ICP development is essentially about promoting change and no change can be achieved without the support of all individuals involved. There are a number of approaches to managing the human dimensions of change and this is a brief introduction of some of the approaches to involving staff in the change process.[1]

Most people do not like change. Implementing change successfully often means working with people who would prefer things to continue as they are.

Top Down Verses Bottom Up
Change can be imposed by senior management or it can develop from below. Top down change will usually have a clear plan, will have support and leadership and will have clear objectives. However, staff may see the change process as an imposition from above and may be less likely to feel part of the process. Bottom up change will be more inclusive of staff, because this is change from 'within the ranks'. It is likely to be a continuous, rather than an episodic process. There is often no plan or clear objective to the change; outcomes may not be supported by senior management as they may not fit with organisational objectives and senior management acceptance of solutions may be less likely.

The best option is a combination of the two approaches. Clear leadership and support for the process from senior management, with clear objectives. Staff should be using improvement tools in their daily work and change should be a continuous process.

Change will be encouraged by 'intelligent leadership'[2]. Clinicians are more likely to become involved in change if they are confident that managers understand the problems faced by the service and are competent in the understanding and analysis of data.

The Four Essential Factors
Before staff will embrace change, four factors must be present.

■ **Dissatisfaction:** Staff must be unhappy with the process as it currently is. No one will want to change something that is working well.

■ **Vision:** There must be a view that things can be better and an agreed vision of how things could be. We do not give up what we have without a clear idea of what we will have in its place.

1 *Further information can be found in A Guide to Good Practice: Elective Services* (NLIAH 2005) *and the Improvement Leadership Guide updated Box Set* (Modernisation Agency 2005)

2 *Intelligent Leadership* Alistair Mant, 1999 ISBN 1865180527

- **Capacity:** There must be capacity to change. There must be a commitment from senior management to change processes and to provide the resources that will be necessary to implement the change.

- **First Steps:** There must be a clear understanding by all of what will happen first. Overcoming inertia is easier if there is a clear plan, with manageable first steps.

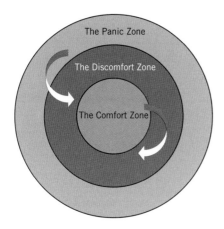

The Comfort Zone
Part of involving people is getting them out of that comfort zone where they feel that the status quo is acceptable. However, it must be done in such a way that staff do not panic. In any group there will be those in the comfort zone ("I don't want to change!") and those in the panic zone ("I can't change!"). The art is in moving both groups into the discomfort zone ("I can change!").

What is in it for me?
The best way to move people forward is to identify what is in the change process for them. Everyone will have some motivation for either adopting or resisting change. Everyone will have something about the current process that they do not like. The key to good change management is to identify and use these drivers. If you ensure that solutions to problems meet the needs of the staff, they will be much easier to implement.

Transitions
"Every beginning ends something."
Paul Valery, French Poet

Every change destroys something that has gone before and some people will regret that loss even if they are happy with the new process. William Bridges[2] calls the process that people go through as they face change 'transition'. Transitions starts with an ending, go through a period of uncertainty and end with a new beginning.

- **Managing the Ending:** Before you can start something new, you must end what used to be. To do this effectively you must understand who is losing what, and what over? You must positively acknowledge the losses and be clear what is over and what is not. It is often useful to mark endings. In some cases, you can let people take a bit of the past with them – their door sign, their desk, a plant or poster.

- **Managing a Neutral Zone:** Neither the old ways nor the new ways seems to be working. This is the dangerous time, where anxiety rises and motivation falls. There will be more illness, but it will also be a more creative time; redefine it and use it constructively. Create temporary systems to work through this stage.

- **A New Beginning:** This is the easy part, especially if the ending has been managed effectively. You must clarify and communicate the purpose, painting a picture of how it will be. Create a plan and show everyone their part in the future.

2 *Managing Transitions: Making sense of Life's Changes*. William Bridges, 1981
ISBN 0201000822

In order to make the most appropriate and effective changes the Modernisation Agency in England developed a series of information guides and tools, published as a boxed set of manuals (see page 14). See also the *Guide to Good Practice (Elective Care)* published by the NLIAH, chapter 9.

Developing an Integrated Care Pathway

2

The Development Tools

Base Line Audit

The ICP development team must gather all evidence needed to underpin the ICP. Consider the need for base line audit of current practice. This will enable evaluation of the ICPs success.

> **Gwent Stroke Project Focus Group**
> An example of the use of a focus group to aid service improvement within the development of a Stroke Integrated Care Pathway
>
> Gwent stroke project set up a series of focus groups to gather the consensus opinion on what changes were required to ensure improvement in service delivery by the teams in primary care.
>
> The task was to focus and reach agreement on the desired outcomes, based on the best available evidence. The main areas where improvements could be made were very similar in all six groups in this project The learning day was felt to have been of benefit in that there was a vast amount of 'sharing ideas' across different teams.

Patient/Staff Questionnaire

Using questions can identify doubts and fears which can unlock the process and give the ICP development team an opportunity to find solutions before problems become insurmountable.

Focus Groups

Focus groups involve small groups of service users, encompassing both staff, patients and carers who have experience of the service. The decision on how many times the group meets will be dependent on the questions and findings to be gleaned.

The improvements should be **SMART** (specific, measurable, achievable, realistic and results centered, and time bound) objectives.

Blue Skies Thinking

This exercise is a powerful technique for generating literally hundreds of ideas in relation to a particular problem. It works through the interaction of a small group of people who are given the permission to voice even the most absurd ideas. Often, the best ideas are sparked off by something ridiculous.

These exercises should take place somewhere with plenty of space and no distractions and require a facilitator and a recorder. They are broken down into two stages:

Stage 1

A free-ranging generation of as many ideas as possible, with the facilitator ensuring that the five rules of are followed:

■ Address one problem at a time

■ No criticism allowed because no idea is too ridiculous

■ Wild ideas are encouraged

■ Ideas sparked by ideas are encouraged

■ Quantity rather than quality

Stage 2

Filter through the list of ideas for the best ones, group those that work together, and rank the best ones for further discussion.

Groups should ideally consist of between six and ten people. Good facilitation is essential to keep up the momentum of the session and to the participation of all members of the group. Sessions should generally not run for longer than an hour, with the ideas generation stage on one particular problem lasting no more than 15 minutes .

PDSA Cycles

After analysis and identification of the problems comes the moment of truth; what can be done to improve the service? How can change be introduced in a clinical environment so that staff feel comfortable and patient care is improved not disrupted? Traditionally, the NHS approach to change has been through project management. Project plans are produced, Gantt charts prepared, programmes of meetings are arranged, change is introduced, but then the project meets opposition and does not always succeed.

NLIAH recommends an alternative approach to introducing change. A process of continuous improvement through incremental changes; the use of PDSA (plan, do study act) cycles provides a model of improvement that enables an ongoing change programme to exist in a clinical environment.

What is the PDSA model?

The model for improvement has two parts: it starts with three questions, followed by a series of improvement cycles.

1. **What are we trying to accomplish?**
    The start of the improvement process should be a statement of the aims of the project. It is impossible to reach a goal without knowing what it is. The goal statement should be clear, specific, aspirational and measurable.

2. **How will we know that a change is an improvement?**
    The key to an effective improvement process is measurement. Without effective measures there is no way to know whether any change is improving the process. A range of measures for improvement is central to any improvement process.

3. **What changes can we make that will result in improvement?**
    The PDSA cycles are a way of testing suggested improvements in a controlled environment. The changes that are developed in response to question three are the changes that the cycles will test. Changes can come from staff suggestion, from other sites that have looked at the same problems or from literature

The Cycle

The PDSA cycle is a repeated cycle of four stages.

- **Plan:** Define the question that you want answered in this phase, including what you would expect the outcome to be. Design an experiment to test the question, covering the 'who, what, when and how' of the cycle and the measures that will be used to determine success.

- **Do:** Do the experiment, ensuring the data is being collected. Record what went wrong and what went well. Were there any unexpected outcomes?

- **Study:** Get everyone together to look at the data. What has been learned? Do the outcomes agree with the predictions? Are there circumstances where the outcome might be different?

- **Act:** Decide what to do in the next cycle. Should the change be implemented more widely? Can it be extended to more patients or is something else necessary? What will be the objective of the next cycle? If the change was unsuccessful, it should be abandoned and something different tried for the next Cycle; there should not be pressure to adopt every change.

> **Using 'Plan Do Study Act' Cycles in Endoscopy**
> **Cardiff and Vale NHS Trust**
> Demand and Capacity principals were applied to Endoscopy services at the University Hospital of Wales. Detailed process mapping at multi-disciplinary workshops identified opportunities to improve patient preparation prior to the endoscopy examination as a means of increasing the number of patients who attended.
>
> The team planned a PDSA cycle by selecting an Endoscopy list for non-urgent patients and training a senior nurse to carry out telephone pre-admission assessment of patients. Data collected included changes in patient attendance rates and the time taken to assess the patient before and after implementing the service.
>
> On completion of the PDSA cycle the nurse-led pre-admission service was shown to have achieved a reduction in patients' non-attendance or cancellation rate from 18% to 6%, which if made available to all patients, could increase patient attendances by up to 500 a year.

A series of cycles

Improvement is the result of a continuing series of cycles building on previous results. Each PDSA cycle is short, making small improvements to the status quo. The result is a steady improvement in process over time. One 'ramp' of cycles relating to one process may be undertaken in parallel with another series dealing with a different problem but the key is to have a series of changes, made in a systematic way, where the results from each cycle are available.

The PDSA model is ideally suited to introducing change in a complex clinical environment, where there is a high element of risk. Small changes are more acceptable to staff and patients and there is far less disruptions than the more traditional 'major redesign programme'. The process also promotes the philosophy that change is a normal continuous process that the staff are involved in, rather than a major event that 'happens to' people.

GP feedback systems

The use of access protocols in primary care is a common way of trying to reduce demand on secondary care services. NLIAH recommends an alternative to access protocols; the use of active feedback to GPs.

Discovery Interviews

Discovery interviews are used widely by the Modernisation Agency and are a way to explore the impact of illness on patients' everyday lives during each stage of their journey through the health care system.

Process Mapping

One way to process map is to allow the clinical team to plot their individual part in the patient journey using post it notes and a large roll of brown paper. Further information about process mapping can be found in the Guide to Good Practice: Elective Services, as well as later in this Guide (page 24).

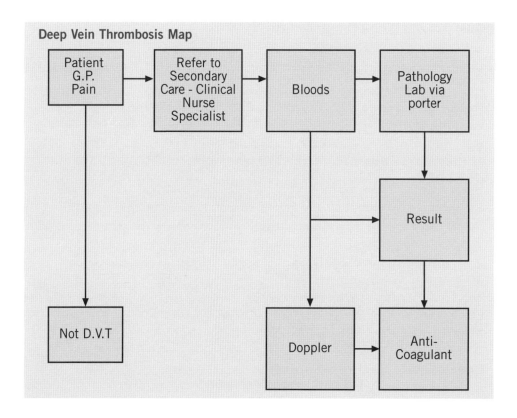

Deep Vein Thrombosis Map

SWOT Fishbone

Within the design process, a SWOT (strengths, weaknesses, opportunities, threats) analysis is often most valuable as a way of evaluating different courses of action.

The fishbone diagram is a useful tool for identifying the constituent parts of a problem and the people, department or other factors that have a bearing on it. It can be used during a meeting to capture and position information or as a means of presenting key issues stemming from an identified problem. It is particularly useful for spotting blockages or successes to progress.

You start by setting out the problem on the left of the spine, then identify all the different factors influencing and contributing to the problem. Once all the factors have been identified they can be explored in turn to see where the real cause of the problem lies. This may mean extending the diagram so that each main cause is broken down into its own possible contributing causes. A prioritised action plan can then be put together which determines the requirements of the ICP.

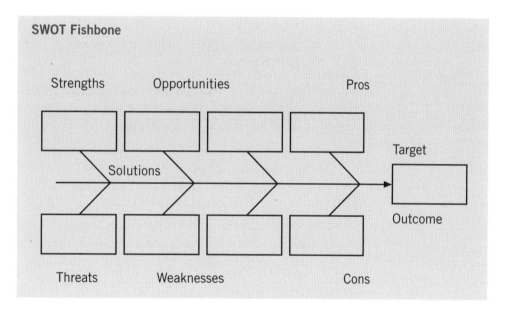

SWOT Fishbone

Strengths · Opportunities · Pros · Target · Solutions · Outcome · Threats · Weaknesses · Cons

Balanced Scorecard

The balance scorecard enables organisations to assess where they sit in the eyes of their customer and how ready they are to meet the challenges they may face to allow them to be considered one of the top providers. If they have already achieved this rating, they need to ensure that they are equipped to sustain their position at the top. The four quadrants of the balance scorecard can assist an organisation in assessing this, can individually support the improvement and development process and can link with other quadrants to support the process.

Customer needs	Organisational needs
Do you know what your customer wants?	Can we supply what the customer wants
Value	**Staff needs**
Are we doing this in a cost effective way, have we adopted the best possible delivery method to address everyone's needs and eliminated unnecessary waste?	Are our staff equipped to deliver (and this covers the knowledge and skills area, as well as being given the tools required) what the customer wants, needs and expects

This is a very simplistic view of the balance scorecard, but if we look at the four quadrants and relate these to health care delivery perhaps it would present a slightly different view.

- **Customer needs:** What do our patients want? How do they want it delivered?

- **Organisation needs:** How can we best meet the needs of the patient? Are we considering the patient when we develop a process or standard of care, or are we simply delivering what 'we feel' is best?

- **Staff needs:** Do we invest in our staff? An organisations' staff are often highly capable and qualified individuals and reinvestment is essential in the recruitment and retention process. If we reinvest, are we just creating a 'knowledge bank'? Reinvestment in staff can assist the organisation in meeting the needs of the patient and ultimately the needs of the organisation itself.

- **Value:** In today's day and age, we need to ensure that as well as providing effective healthcare, that healthcare must also be efficient (meaning timely and valuable). Whilst money does not equate to health, we accept that inefficiency, delay and ineffectiveness can be attributed to waste and waste will equate to cost.

In healthcare, if we take a process and measure it against the four quadrants, it should be quite easy to see in which areas we are performing well and in which areas we need to perform better.

Timeline and Gantt Chart

Henry Laurence Gantt (1861-1919) was a mechanical engineer, management consultant and industry advisor who developed the timeline and Gantt chart as a visual tool to show scheduled and actual progress of projects in the 1920s. They are accepted as a commonplace project management tool today and can be used for the simplest or most complex of projects.

Gantt charts are useful tools for planning and scheduling projects

- Allow you to assess how long a project should take

- Lay out the order in which tasks need to be carried out.

- Help manage the dependencies between tasks.

- Determine the resources needed

Gantt charts are useful tools when a project is under way. They allow you to
- Monitor progress. You can immediately see what should have been achieved at a point in time.

- See how remedial action may bring the project back on course.

The vertical table lists information about each project task and the horizontal bar chart shows tasks durations and start and finish dates on a timescale. The relative positions of the Gantt bar show which tasks are planned to come before or after or overlap the various tasks listed. In addition, personnel and other resources can be assigned to each task in order to ensure the resources are used as efficiently as possible. The Gantt chart can be used throughout the ICP project to track progress by comparing baseline and actual start and finish dates and by checking the percentage of each task that is complete.

The ICP Project Gantt Chart, which can be found at Appendix 3, can be added to throughout the project, as the detailed actions and milestones for each phase are planned. It may include:

■ The main phases

■ Actions and milestones

Each action and milestones will have associated:

■ Timescales

■ Personnel responsible

■ Resources required

For a detailed review of project management see the *Guide to Good Practice (Elective Care)* chapter 7.

2.1 Developing your Integrated Care Pathway

There are eight stages involved in the development of an ICP.

1 - Deciding on an Integrated Care Pathway to Develop

Your clinical area may already be clear about which ICP it needs to develop or it may have several priority areas and clarity needs to be sought. Whichever category your clinical area falls into, it can be helpful to identify all potential areas for ICP development and gain joint agreement from multi-disciplinary teams as to their priority. The organisation's clinical governance and modernisation teams would be able to provide advice regarding priority areas. Priority areas may be identified through:

National Priorities
- National Service Frameworks
- Modernisation Programme Streams
- NICE Guidelines
- Royal College Guidelines
- Audit Commission Reports
- National Research
- Welsh Assembly Government performance targets

Local Priorities
- High volume
- High cost
- High risk
- Areas where there is significant variation in practice
- Complaints – lessons learnt

Once you have selected an ICP for development, it is essential that you contact the person who has overall responsibility for ICP development within your organisation who will register this development work and advise you.

1 - Deciding on an ICP to Develop

2 - Identifying Stakeholders and Leads

3 - Identifying Lead and Team Responsibilities

4 - Process Mapping

5 - Initial Audit and Data Collection

6 - ICP Content Development

7 - Pilot and Implementation

8 - Regular Review of the ICP

2 - Identifying Stakeholders and Leads

A stakeholder is anyone who may have an interest in the ICP or its outcomes. Stakeholders may therefore be identified under two categories: those who need to be directly involved in the development of the ICP (internal stakeholders); and those for whom a consultation exercise would be appropriate (external stakeholders). Stakeholders require a clear mechanism through which they can ask questions, feedback and give ideas or express concerns. It is better to address these issues early in the process than to wait until the implementation stage, when the ICP itself could be undermined.

Directly Involved (internal stakeholders)

- User, e.g. patients, carers, advocacy services
- ICP project team staff
- Referrers
- Relevant Departments e.g. Clinical Governance, IM and T
- Other Agencies
- Specialist Services
- Other Organisations
- The Multi Disciplinary Teams
- Primary Care

Indirectly Involved (external stakeholders)

- Trust Boards
- Medical Advisory Committee
- Nursing Advisory Group
- Social Services
- Voluntary associations

3 - Identifying Lead and Team Responsibilities

ICP Team Lead: As well as identifying stakeholders, it is also crucial to establish a team lead or champion for the ICP, to drive and sustain the change process. The lead's remit will be to:

- Identify representatives to form an ICP Team

- Lead and motivate the team in writing the ICP according to the strategic approach across the health and social care community

- Support the team in identifying the key variances which will need to be tracked within the ICP

- Ensure evidence based best practice (EBBP) is embedded in the development of the ICP

- Identify, plan and assist in the delivery of changes associated with the ICP implementation

- Represent the views of the ICP Team in all aspects of the specific ICP development and implementation including successful and problematic areas

- Share information on the development on the ICP across the health community

- To be involved in the implementation of the ICP across the specialty areas

ICP Team: For the authorising or senior development team, choose motivated individuals from the suggested list of directly involved stakeholders. The team's remit will be to:

- Represent the views and requirements of the patient and service in all aspects of the ICP

- Identify, plan and assist in the delivery of benefits associated with the implementation of the ICP

- Identify the activities from the patient journey that will be included in the ICP

- Identify problematic areas across the ICP

- Promote communication regarding the ICP across the immediate working area and the wider organisation

- Highlight any issues or concerns to the Team Lead

4 - Process Mapping

As ICPs are tools for improving care delivered to patients, then it follows that in order to make improvements, a firm understanding of what is actually happening is captured, understood and analysed by the whole clinical team, key stakeholders and patients from the outset.

One of the most effective methods suggested for teams to begin understanding the processes which makes up the complete patient journey and their experience along the way, is to undertake a 'process mapping' exercise.

Process mapping can produce a 'map' of the patient's journey from their perspective. From this map, the multi-disciplinary team can learn to appreciate the real problems in the system and identify the fundamental improvements needed that will have the biggest positive impact for patients and staff.

A process map is essentially a picture of the activities or tasks that over time deliver a product, outcome or achieves a desired condition. It is a high level view of an overall process showing the main sub processes and their interrelationships.

The map will help to define:

- The sequence of steps and activities performed

- Specific responsibilities for these steps and activities

- Areas that lie outside the process but impact on it

- The relationships that exist between the different professionals in the process

- Potential problem areas

It may be helpful for the ICP development team to set ground rules before the start of the exercise and emphasise that process mapping is about trying to really understand the patient's experience at various stages of their journey and not about blame for hold-ups or delays. Developing the map from the point of view of a clearly defined group of patients will keep the exercise focussed and productive.

A process mapping sessions of the patient's journey should give the team:

■ A key starting point from which to identify improvements.

■ The opportunity to bring together multi-disciplinary teams from primary, secondary and tertiary settings, health and social care and most importantly, patients and carers.

■ An overview of the whole process, often for the first time.

■ An aid to effectively planning where to test improvement ideas; where they are likely to have the most impact.

■ Brilliant ideas, from staff that really know the system and how it works.

■ An interactive event involving 'everyone'.

■ An end product – the map, which is clear and visible.

Having undertaken process mapping, the team will be able to begin evaluating their practice against current best practice and begin asking themselves questions about the appropriateness of certain activities, tasks or investigations. Here opportunities for improvement are identified and changes in practice can begin to be discussed and agreed.[1]

In this context ICPs can easily be viewed as a logical method of incorporating clinical effectiveness into practice and from this position the team can begin to determine how the process mapping information can be translated into the first draft of the ICP.

An example: A surgical ICP could be developed in the following sections:

■ Primary care initial management

■ pre-operative assessment

■ in-patient stay

■ out-patient care

■ primary care management on discharge from acute services.

Each part or section could be developed contemporaneously to form the whole journey.

1 *Middleton & Roberts (2003). Integrated Care Pathways: A Practical Approach to Implementation*

5 - Initial Audit and Data Collection

The baseline audit for an ICP is undertaken at the beginning of the project. The results will not only indicate where there are gaps in the service but also to what extent standards are currently being met. The audit will also form the basis of the evaluation of the ICP, as initial data can be compared with end of pilot data.

The steps involved in a baseline audit project are:

1. **Form an Audit Team:** Which members of the ICP team are best placed to undertake this piece of work? A multi-disciplinary team will be able to give a good perspective on what data is required and how to identify it within the notes. The team may decide that it would be appropriate to consult patients in planning the project; if so you may need to obtain ethical approval.
It is important that colleagues in positions of authority support the project and have the commitment to see changes put into practice.

2. **Decide on the Standards:** Your ICP will be based on national or local standards or consensus/custom based best practice or a combination of all three. It is crucial to measure key milestones or actions against appropriate standards so that the evaluation audit will be consistent.

3. **Select an Audit Sample:** The team should agree whether to audit over a given period of time or choose a sample size from the patient population. There are ways of selecting samples of patients which you can be satisfied are representative of the larger group. Gathering data from an appropriate sample group is important as you must ensure that your data is robust for your team to base decisions on. Your local audit facilitator can give you more advice about choosing your sample.

4. **Decide What Data to Collect:** Is your audit going to be retrospective or concurrent? Is data going to be collected using an audit form or entered directly onto a computer? A small pilot audit will ensure that your data collection tool works, especially if a team is collecting the data. The pilot may reveal that some of your questions are ambiguous, that the form is difficult to complete or that you are simply not getting the information you want. Ensure you allow sufficient time for data collection and modification of your initial data collection tool.

5. **Collect the Data:** You have planned every detail of your audit and you are ready to go; collect your data. Make sure you are clear about exactly who is going to be responsible for doing what and when.

6. **Analyse the Data:** Pull your data together in the most meaningful way and compare your results against your standards.

7. **Present your Findings:** Present your findings to colleagues and agree an action plan of the way forward. The results will assist you in deciding any service re-design that is required at this stage of the ICP development.

8. **Evaluate your Findings:** The baseline audit can clarify how to move forward but can also form an indicator of the success of the ICP. Once the ICP is complete and implemented an infrastructure for continuous improvement should be put in place to consistently measure the performance of the ICP and the attainment of the standards.

6 - Integrated Care Pathway Content Development

An ICP should contain:

- Activities: These are the planned elements of care contained in the process. They are based upon EBBP

- Detail: Any tools or descriptions already required in the case notes, including observations, fluid balance charts, demographic details etc

- Outcomes: These can range from clinical outcomes (tests etc) to process outcomes (e.g. standards achieved to targets) and may include patient or staff outcomes

- Variance Tracking: The unique element of an ICP that allows planned and actual care to be compared, leading to continuous improvement of practice

Principles of design and layout

The clinical content of an ICP cannot be dictated; this will be determined by the team with expertise in managing that particular group of patients, for whom the document is designed. However, standards for design and layout can be recommended and are found at Appendix 2.

7 - Pilot and Implementation

Communication and Education Plan

A robust communication and education plan is essential to underpin a successful ICP Project. The purpose of communication and education is to ensure that appropriate messages are delivered to the appropriate people in the most appropriate manner at the most appropriate time and in the most appropriate place. Also, that the key stakeholders are directly involved or consulted appropriately.

A variety of communication methods will be used to disseminate information about the project. The nature of the information will change as the project develops. Ongoing advice and support will be available throughout the project from the ICP development team. This will include general awareness raising about the concept of ICPs and the approach taken locally. When nearing the implementation stage, the focus will be on ensuring that all areas are aware of how the ICP will impact on their work, including the opportunities and challenges presented. Immediately prior to and during implementation, training and user feedback will form the main communication strategy building on the methods employed earlier in the project. Each organisation has forums and clinical teams, which will form essential communication and education networks for dissemination of progress and ensuring involvement and feedback from future ICP users.

Implementation

As for any process of change, careful preparation needs to be made for the implementation of the ICP. This preparation should begin sometime before the ICP documentation is ready for use, when the wider clinical team needs to be made aware of the developments that are taking place. The appearance of the ICP in the clinical area should not come as a shock.

To effectively implement the ICP, consideration should be given to the following:

■ Identify the pilot site for the ICP and the date for the launch of the new documentation

■ Inform staff in the area prior to the launch date, circulate copies of the ICP so staff are familiar with the layout. Notices can be used to increase awareness

■ Arrange training sessions for all staff who will come into contact with the ICP; this will involve going through a copy of the documentation, explaining its purpose and how it should be completed, especially the recording of variances

■ Pilot the ICP for a defined period of time or for a defined number of cases: this will depend on the patient group for whom the ICP has been developed (i.e. high volume or not)

■ Ensure that copies of the ICP are kept in an accessible place and that staff know where to find them (e.g. in a clearly labelled open box)

■ Put a 'comments/communication sheet' or a staff satisfaction survey near the spare copies of the ICP in the clinical area so any queries, comments or issues can be noted. This may be available from your local ICP Manager, audit department or public and patient involvement lead

Development of the ICP and the pilot period is time consuming; once the evaluation of the pilot has taken place and the appropriate amendments have been made, the ICP can be put into use on a more permanent basis and the more intense work comes to an end.

Remember when piloting/implementing the ICP:

■ There should be support to local clinical leads to deliver ICP training to staff involved in the pilot

■ There should be senior management support for each local ICP for the first week of implementation

■ The high profile of the ICP should be maintained throughout the pilot period

■ There should be a re-launch of the ICP when it has been amended and updated, including publicity and feedback from the pilot

■ The pilot versions of the ICP should be removed and replaced with the updated version

For long-term implementation, remember:

■ There must be a regular variance tracking feedback session incorporated into routine educational/team sessions. It is this that will prevent the 'fizzling out' syndrome that projects can be prone to.

8 - Regular Review of the ICP

When reviewing the ICP, you should focus on three particular questions;

■ **Completion of the ICP:** is it being used in all appropriate cases? How is it being completed? What information is being omitted? Are staff using conventional record keeping in addition/instead of the ICP?

■ **Types of Variances Recorded:** have any been recorded? If so, are they appropriate; is it clear that staff know what variances are and how to record them?

■ **Staff satisfaction:** has the generic questionnaire been completed? What trends does analysis show, if any?

Review of the ICP is very much an ongoing process. After the pilot phase, things tend to settle down as the new version is launched for a longer period of time. The ICP is a dynamic tool which needs to be reviewed and amended as part of the ongoing audit process; the frequency of review depends on the variances recorded. Variance recording allows any variation from the expected plan of care to be monitored to ensure that the ICP continues to develop and meet the changing needs of the patient group it was designed for.

The development of ICPs is by no means simple but the process can be streamlined by adopting a structured approach.

The four meeting model described here condenses the principles set out in 2.1 to a short timescale. This approach has been used in Trusts to develop a number of basic ICPs quickly.

The ICP development structure can take the form of four meetings in which particular elements are covered. Before every meeting, preparatory work will need to be conducted by the key members of the development team to create a platform from which to base the agenda of the following meeting. The diagram below explains the model. Detailed descriptions and examples of the sub-steps can be found below.

1

Meeting 1 Preparation

1.1 Before the first meeting: Collect baseline data on patient/condition on which the ICP will focus

Meeting 1

1.2 Explain to the team what an ICP is and have a copy of an extant ICP of the specialty available

1.3 Develop a high level patient flow process map

1.4 Identify where the ICP will start and finish

1.5 Identify the stages of care in the ICP

1.6 Identify the patient discharge criteria

1.7 Identify the perceived problems with the current care

2

Meeting 2 Preparation

2.1   Before Meeting 2: Each member of the team to confirm discharge criteria with wider colleague circle and to do the same for the perceived problems with the current care

Meeting 2

2.2   Confirm perceived problems with the current care

2.3   Decide how to identify if perceived problems really 'are' problems

2.4   Develop a plan for collecting sample data to identify if perceived problems really 'are' problems

2.5   Develop an initial list of 'ultimate patient outcomes' that the ICP needs to focus on

3

Meeting 3 Preparation

3.1   Before Meeting 3: Each professional within the team to identify their particular areas of responsibility within each stage of the ICP

Meeting 3

3.2   Professionals to present back to the team their particular areas of responsibility

3.3   Presentation of the confirmed problems with the current care

3.4   Identify how to minimise the problems

3.5   Determine the criteria patients must meet to pass through the discreet stages of the ICP

4

Meeting 4 Preparation

4.1   Each member to develop a final list of individual professionals' inputs and patient outcomes/expectations

4.2   One member to develop draft clinical and patient versions of ICP and distribute

Meeting 4

4.3   Review the draft ICP and agree final amendments

4.4   Identify ICP and team's ability to deliver on agreed outcomes

4.5   Develop a plan for the ICP pilot phase

4.6   Set up a variance tracking database

The Four Meeting Model: Sub-Step Descriptions and Examples

1

Ref.	Action	Explanation
1.1	**Before the first meeting:** Collect baseline data on patient/condition on which the ICP will focus (including outcomes).	Once you have decided what ICP to develop and what patients group to focus on, you need to gather data to inform the ICP such as Average Length of Stay (ALOS), type of admission, discharge destination, date of surgery etc. This information will illustrate the variation within current practice attributable to either the patient or clinical care.
1.2	Explain to the team what an ICP is and have a copy of an extant ICP of the specialty available	Everyone who will be expected to use the ICP needs to know what it is. Use the ICP to see what others are doing and to identify how your ICP will need to be different.
1.3	Develop a high level patient flow process map	Using process mapping methodology, gather the relevant people into a room and develop your high level process map. This is the perfect opportunity to give professionals a chance to see the current process from the patients' perspective and take out steps which do not add value to patient care.
1.4	Identify where the ICP will start and finish	The ICP has to have a clear beginning and end. This may be the moment patients enter the GP surgery to entering the hospital or entering ITU to discharge. It is easier to develop an ICP within one organisation rather than to develop across organisational boundaries but it is feasible to do so.
1.5	Identify the stages of care in the ICP	Within an ICP, there will be discreet stages of care e.g., assessment, post surgical, discharge. Identify these stages so that the ICP development is more focused and does not appear so daunting.
1.6	Identify the patient discharge criteria	From the outset, you need to have clear ideas about what the patient discharge criteria are. Identifying the discharge destination and working back can assist in identifying discharge criteria. Criteria should include physical, domestic, social and transport planning, e.g. is the patient happy to go home, does the patient have transport to take them home?
1.7	Identify the perceived problems with the current care	It is likely that within the current system there are problems. Identify what you think these problems are.

2

Ref.	Action	Explanation
2.1	**Before Meeting 2:** Each member of the team to confirm discharge criteria with wider colleague circle and to do the same for the perceived problems with the current care	After the first meeting, all the members need to go away and talk to their specialty colleagues to get a consensus on whether the discharge criteria and the perceived problems which the group has come up with are suitable and actually perceived.
2.2	Confirm perceived problems with the current care	In the team, you need to discuss the perceived problems as discussed and agreed in your specialty areas.
2.3/2.4	Decide how to identify if perceived problems really 'are' problems and develop a plan for collecting sample data to identify if perceived problems really 'are' problems	Once you have a list of perceived problems, you need to develop a plan to identify whether they really are problems. This will probably involve collecting data from notes or developing a data collection exercise to run for a few weeks. Keep the data collection exercise small, e.g. medical records of the last 10 admitted patients.
2.5	Develop an initial list of 'ultimate patient outcomes' that the ICP needs to focus on	Based on the variations in care (linked to 1.1) and perceived problems (linked to 1.7, 2.3, 2.4), identify the best practice patient focused aims which the ICP needs to focus on, e.g. 70% of patients can go home in 3 days.

3

Ref.	Action	Explanation
3.1	**Before Meeting 3:** Each professional within the team to identify their particular areas of responsibility within each stage of the ICP	Linking to 1.5, the members of the group now need to look in detail at the sections within the ICP which are particularly pertinent to them and for which they have responsibility, such as nursing, clerking, discharge. The group needs to refer to the good practice evidence available and record relevant references.
3.2	Professionals to present back to the team their particular areas of responsibility	Once members of the team have had an opportunity to discus their responsibilities with specialty colleagues, these findings need to be fed back to the team.
3.3	Presentation of the confirmed problems with the current care	The team needs to discuss the original perceived problems, as previously discussed with colleagues, in light of the data collection exercise (linked to 3.1). A list of confirmed actual problems needs to be drawn up.

3.4	Identify how to minimise the problems	The group needs to confirm that the actual problems which can not be addressed prior to the ICP implementation, will be addresses within the ICP plan of care. It may be necessary to develop new strategies in the plan to address the problems e.g. add in additional care plan for patients with diabetes.
3.5	Determine the criteria patients must meet to pass through the discreet stages of the ICP	Determine the interim goals the patient needs to attain to pass through the discreet stages within the ICP. This may mean 'patient is able to walk unaided' and therefore can pass to the discharge section.

4

Ref.	Action	Explanation
4.1	**Before Meeting 4:** Each member to develop a final list of individual professionals' inputs and patient outcomes/ expectations	The draft lists of patient outcomes and staff responsibilities need to be forwarded to the member of the team collating the information.
4.2	**Before Meeting 4:** One member to develop draft clinical and patient version of ICP and distribute	One member of the team needs to put all of the information together and write the draft ICP. ICPs need to focus on patient outcomes. Draw up a draft list of these outcomes, e.g. rather than having an aim of 'nurse supports patient to sit in chair', think about 'patient is able to sit in chair with support'. The ICP is not about the nurse but the patient. If your organisation has decided to adopt a patient version of the ICP, this would also be the time to write a draft version.
4.3	Review the draft ICP and agree final amendments	In the final meeting, the team needs to go through the draft ICP and agree the final version. If this does not happen now, there is a danger that the ICP will continue to be modified and amended and never become 'live'.
4.4	Identify ICP and team's ability to deliver on agreed outcomes	The group needs to confirm that the care plan within the ICP does minimise actual problems (linking to 3.4, 3.5) and maximises the ICP and the clinical teams' ability to deliver on the ICPs patient focused aims (linked to 2.5).

4.5	Develop a plan for the ICP pilot phase	The pilot phase needs to be planned. You need to decide who will conduct the initial training. It is useful to have a combination of training styles such as seminars, one-to-one meetings etc. Rather than focusing on a specified time to conduct the pilot, it will be more useful to identify a specific number of ICPs/patients, maybe 10.
4.6	Set up a variance tracking database	In order to make the best use of the variances, you need to develop a variance tracking database. This may be developed by your department, trust or may be a manual system. NLIAH has developed a basic database which you may find useful to use. The best analysis will be gained by collecting variance data from patients at the time that the variance occurs, rather than in retrospect; this minimises work and the possibility of data being lost or forgotten. It is important that variance data is collected for each patient otherwise the team will not gain adequate feedback on what is happening with the guidelines in the pathways.

Once the ICP has been developed it is very important to ensure that the momentum for using the ICP is maintained. This can be supported by organising a post-pilot review meeting which will identify what problems were encountered during the ICP implementation phase. During this meeting, a team will need to be established to regularly review the ICP and any variances. Subsequently, the ICP review team should meet regularly and if necessary establish small working parties to look at particular trends detected by variance tracking and identify whether processes or care requires improvement (see also the table on page 28).

3

Variances and Variance Tracking

ICPs offer a structure for care delivery, they do not replace individual practitioner clinical judgement and are not a substitute for clinical judgement. Not all patients will follow a predictable ICP. Any professional may and should deviate from the ICP provided they have a valid reason for doing so; the intent is for clinical freedom to be exercised according to individual patient need. In ICP terms, this is termed a 'variance'.

Variances occur when what is expected to happen does not. Variances are then recorded by the professional, noting why the decision was made and what remedial or alternative action was taken . This is known as 'variance tracking'

Johnson (1997)[1] explores the importance of variance within her definition of ICPs: 'An ICP amalgamates all the anticipated elements of care and treatment of all members of the multidisciplinary team, for a patient or client of a particular case-type or grouping within an agreed time frame, for the achievement of agreed outcomes. Any deviation from the plan is documented as a 'variance', the analysis of which provides information for the review of current practice'

Wales[2] builds on this to say that the unique element of the ICP tool that distinguishes it from any previous care planning and care management tools is the recording, tracking and analysing of variances to improve care and the ICP. Therefore, if there is no variance tracking mechanism you are not truly using an ICP. Variance tracking is the tool that takes ICPs a step further than other care planning techniques.

The method by which variances are documented may vary throughout organisations, many of which have previously implemented widespread documentation redesign for each ICP. An alternative method being explored by one Welsh Trust is to utilise current documentation, while providing individual clinical teams with the tools necessary to draw upon current evidence based best practice. This is done through process mapping the status quo, formulating a set of sequentially numbered ICP notes, developing a précised numerical flowchart and utilising a generic variance tracking record which accompanies all ICPs.

1 *Johnson (1997) Pathways of Care*
Blackwell Science p37

2 *Wales (2003) Integrated Care Pathways -*
What are they or how can they be used?
Clin. Gov. Bulletin 4.2

However variance tracking is undertaken within individual organisations, Shuttleworth (2003)[1] discusses the vital components necessary for structured variance tracking to ensure that all required variances in care are monitored and analysed; she suggests that the method used should be:

■ quick

■ intuitive

■ accessible

■ meaningful

■ part of normal routine record keeping

■ clearly linked to the relevant activity by a unique identifier.

It should not involve the practitioner in time wasting duplication, searching out tracking sheets and working out how to complete them or having to describe in longhand, the activity in question.

For variance tracking to be most useful consideration should be given to the following structure:

■ Is the activity uniquely numbered?

■ Is there a record of date and time?

■ Is there a record of who is completing a particular aspect of care (professional code or text)?

■ Is there a signature record or key within the document to link initials to professionals' full names/designations?

■ Is there a space for recording whether an activity has been undertaken '✔'or not '+' or 'met' or 'unmet'?

■ Is there indication as to what the cause of the variance is (code or text)?

■ Is there a record of what happens as a result of the variation from planned practice (code or text)?

When variance tracking has been audited, trends to identify what has and has not happened can be easily identified. Reasons for deviation from the ICP can be identified; whether this is due to individual clinical judgement, operational or systems failure, including time lapses or blockages in the system or patient choice. The identification of trends can help to manage clinical risk and allow for the evaluation of care provided through the ICP. This information can then be fed back to the individual clinical teams to enable them to establish a clear picture of what is happening and what they may need to do to address training or education deficits or whether they need to revisit the ICP to complete the audit cycle.

1 Shuttleworth, A(ed) Nursing Times Protocol Based Care. Emap Healthcare. London (2003).

4 Continuous Review and Improvement

Sustainability and Continuous Improvement

ICPs provide a systematic approach to the review and implementation of changes and improvements to clinical practice. The ICP model directly empowers the cycle of review, implementation of changes and improvements to practice, directly complementing clinical governance agendas.

ICPs bring to life guidelines and protocols, embedding them into the patient record and using them on a day-to-day basis to ensure that locally agreed standards for best practice are met, or if not met, that the reasons why are highlighted and the action taken is logged. This ensures that patients receive the best evidenced based care possible.

An ICP model consists of a practical solution to completing the cycle of collecting, collating and reviewing information and improving care. It can add to the evidence needed to form the basis of business plans and commissioning and service level agreements, which will truly reflect the needs of the service. It is unique in its ability to remain a clinical tool, whilst providing a powerful source of information for operational and strategic management at all levels.

The best ICPs should embrace patient outcome-orientated standards. This approach assists in the task of ensuring continuous improvements in patient care and challenges processes in terms of the effect that they have on the end result for the patient.

An example of a check list for good ICP design developed by Venture Training and Consultancy Ltd. can be found at Appendix 4.

A useful impact plan and evaluation pro forma can be found at Appendix 5.

The Future of ICPs

The future of ICPs in each health community will depend on commitment from within all elements of the management structure. ICPs are one way of delivering redesign, modernisation and clinical governance agendas; they embrace the principles for good patient experiences.

National Service Frameworks (NSFs) and National Institute of Clinical Effectiveness (NICE) Guideline: ICPs will be essential to support the delivery of emerging NSFs and NICE Guidelines. The NSFs will provide the framework from which to develop ICPs, which can then fit together to form an effective patient journey.

Electronic ICPs: The electronic solution should not detract from the major investment which has already been made in the paper version. Tools for developing electronic ICPs should therefore be flexible, to replicate those ICPs in use. The best way is to design a system with parts, which are generic and can be re-used many times, such as an admission, assessment or a referral for CT scan will feature in many ICPs.

Ross[1] states logical reasons for the promotion of electronic ICP's based on the English approach to 'Informing Healthcare'. Currently, within Wales the 'Informing Healthcare Strategy' is being implemented. It is hoped that this strategy will bridge the gap between single patient records and electronic ICPs.

1 *Ross, 'The British Journal of Healthcare Computing & Information Management'* Feb 2001, Vol 18, No1

4.2

The Birmingham Integrated Care Pathway Appraisal Tool

Birmingham and Black County Strategic Health Authority have funded a project investigating the evaluation and validation of ICPs. The ICP Appraisal tool (ICPAT) is a document which aims to:

- Confirm that the tool developed is an ICP

- Ensure that the mechanism used to develop the ICP is robust

- Ensure that the ICP documentation meets at least the minimum legal requirements for clinical documentation.

61 clinical teams from the UK are taking part in the study to evaluate their own ICPs and this will be published in due course.

For further information contact: The School of Health Sciences, University of Birmingham, Edgbaston, Birmingham, B15 2TT.

Appendices

Appendix 1 Putting Patients at the Centre of Care

Example Patient Journey: GP Surgery – AHPs – Outpatients – Ward – Theatre and Post Op Ward – Community Services – Residential Care

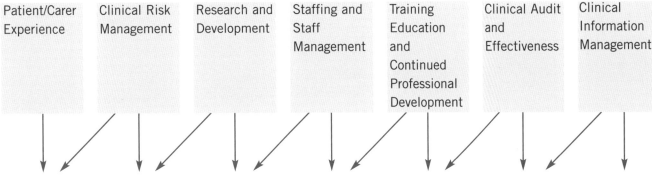

Patient/Carer Experience	Clinical Risk Management	Research and Development	Staffing and Staff Management	Training Education and Continued Professional Development	Clinical Audit and Effectiveness	Clinical Information Management
Patient/Carer involvement in service development and ICP design. Patient held ICPs can be developed; ensuring patient involvement, improved communication, understanding and expectations of standard patient journey, etc.	Identified risks incorporated in ICP e.g. falls risk assessment and falls ICP. Monitoring of ICPs to highlight potential risks to teams.	Evidence Based Practice. Research of current best practice to incorporate into patient journey. Encourages areas of new research.	Involving staff in service development. Support staff to research areas of best practice. ICPs encourage shared knowledge and multi-disciplinary / cross boundary working.	Keep staff up to date with best practice guidelines. Deliver evidence based practice guidelines at the point of care. Involve multi-disciplinary and cross boundary teams in service development.	All ICPs to be audited and reviewed to ensure meeting required standardised best practice. Learning from practice and ensuring service developments as a result of recommendations. Staff Involvement, e.g. multi-disciplinary audits encouraged to span patient journey.	Information to inform service development and thus ICP development. Support audit and changes in practice. Supports staff to monitor practice, identify changes in work flow, etc.

Appendix 1

Appendix 2 Recommendations for Design and Layout

Requirement/Recommendation	Rationale
The ICP should be in an A4 format and remain in the main case notes	This reduces the risk of two documents being available, allows for easier tracking and saves re-filing.
The ICP should be laid out in a table format. Where the lines of the table are not required they may be hidden	Tables facilitate easier formatting and are recognised by web-based programs. The also offer a wide range of possible layouts, within a single document.
Tabs should not be used. Where a tab may have been selected, cells of the table should be split or an indent or bullet may be used	Web-based programs do not recognise tabs.
Font should be Arial preferably point 12 but not smaller than point 10	Arial lends itself to documents of this kind. Print any smaller than this would be difficult to read.
Page numbers should be inserted at the bottom right hand corner of each page. They should be formatted as 'page X of Y'	Page numbers facilitate the use of a contents page, directing multi-disciplinary users straight to the appropriate section and allowing them to identify if any pages are missing.
The cover page should conform to the design and layout demonstrated in the document template. It should include:	**A common format for the outer appearance of the document enables staff from other departments to use and instantly recognise it as an ICP.**
■ The Trust name	To conform to the Trust standard for documents.
■ Patient demographic details, including name, hospital number and date of birth. The space for these details should be designed to allow the use of an addressograph label. The addressograph label should be on every page.	To identify the patient and facilitate filing in the health record. Addressograph labels are instantly recognisable, readable and represent a time-saving method for entering the required information.
■ Allergies must be recorded on the specific alert sheets at the front of the case notes. If necessary allergies may also be recorded on medication sheets within the ICPs	To ensure the patient's safety and avoid unnecessary duplication
■ The title of the ICP together with inclusion criteria	To enable staff to use the ICP for the correct patient group, especially if a section of a larger patient journey.
■ Guidance notes on how to use the ICP. These should be kept to a minimum as the document must be intuitive to use	To provide new users with some simple instruction on the use of the ICP. They should be brief so as not to make them too complex and overwhelming.
■ The name, designation and location of the lead developer of the ICP as a footer	To enable users to return comments on the ICP and its use in practice
■ The version number and date of the last update.	So that users will know when the document is updated and provide an accurate record if care delivery is challenged.
■ Document status, i.e. draft, pilot, operational etc.	So that users can see how established the document is.
■ The C and D ICP reference number, allocated by the ICPs facilitator	For inclusion in a central databases

The following page(s) should be included:

A signature sheet, where each professional making an entry will identify themselves by their name, designation, initials and signature.	A signature sheet allows staff to initial or sign entries without having to enter their name and designation in full. Staff accessing information will be able to identify who has made each entry.
The standard list of approved variance and cause of variance codes, together with any locally agreed codes, specific to this ICP.	Variance codes allow users to enter a number in the event of variance from the ICP, at the time that it occurs. These variance codes provide a structure for live audit and continuous improvement and practice.
A glossary of locally agreed abbreviations, together with any definitions that may be required. These should be terms that are commonly used either in the text of the ICP or that are likely to be used in the free text that the users will enter.	This will facilitate recognition by the users of abbreviations and terms that are used and will allow them to use abbreviations in their entries, instead of entering terms in full. The authors must avoid ambiguity and potential confusion.
The title of the ICP should be included at the top of each page.	To enable easy identification of the document. Should pages become separated they can be reunited with the correct health record.
Name, date of birth and hospital number of the patient must be written on every page of the ICP, preferably in a header.	Should pages become separated they can be reunited with the correct health record.
The ICP should be arranged to reflect the anticipated patient journey. Adjacent to each activity the user should be able to initial to indicate whether the activity has been 'met' or 'not met' and to enter date and time. Variance tracking must be possible either adjacent to the activity, on a separate page or preferably, at the foot of the page. Variance has three distinct elements: variance (recorded as a code) cause of variance (recorded as a code) and action taken (free text). Additional notes may be recorded in the action taken box and should facilitate this. A time, date and initials box should be provided for subsequent action.	The will result in comprehensive record of care and information that can be utilised for audit and continuous improvement purposes.

Structure and Content

The structure of the ICP will be at least partly determined by the clinical content and the requirements of the patient group.	However, the recommendations below will result in a more user friendly document.
The ICP should have a logical flow, being arranged as a chronological record of care. The sequence of events should be clear. Bear in mind that an ICP aims to have: ■ The right people ■ Doing the right things ■ In the right order ■ At the right time ■ In the right place ■ With the right outcome	This will make the ICP more intuitive to use, allowing staff unfamiliar with the patient group to use the ICP and deliver the standard of care as prescribed. This also ensures the most appropriate health professional delivers care at the most appropriate stage.
Clinical content must be linked to accepted good practice, guidelines and protocols.	Ensures that the ICP is a vehicle to implement evidence based best practice.

Guidelines and protocols should only be reproduced in full within an ICP when this is deemed absolutely necessary. Ordinarily the user should be directed to these tools and documents at another location for reference.	Inclusion of all related documents would result in an ICP that was too bulky and difficult to navigate. It must be clear how a team has agreed a technique or method and the user must be able to locate the original evidence. Documents must be written so as to prevent plagiarism.
The clinical content must accurately reflect the anticipated patient journey and expected outcomes.	Otherwise the incidence of variance will be too common and less meaningful.
Whilst the introduction of an ICP may represent an opportunity to improve systems and therefore care, the document must nevertheless be an accurate reflection of realistic expectations.	Otherwise the incidence of variance will be too common and less meaningful.
When recommending referrals to other professionals within an activity always refer to the role, not an individual or their contact details.	Staff and organisational changes could make the ICP obsolete.
When developing the ICP identify the areas where the multi-disciplinary team be duplicating any paperwork and find solutions to avoid this situation occurring within the ICP.	Ineffective duplicating is wasteful of staff and patient time and resource and can lead to inaccurate recording of data.
The activity/action is clear, who is doing it, when.	Activities must be measurable to allow for variances to be tracked.
Wherever appropriate include a standard.	Activities must be measurable to allow for variances to be tracked.
Terms are qualified, e.g. CAHMS referral form NOT referral forms.	To clarify the activity and avoid ambiguity.
Avoid synonyms, abbreviations and jargon	To clarify the activity and avoid ambiguity.
Verbs are used to describe the activities.	To clarify the activity and avoid ambiguity.
EBBP(ebbp) is referenced back to source.	To access full research if required and to assure others that ICP follows EBBP.
Incorporate 'blank' pages in the ICP format to record additional activities and a section if appropriate for recording individual problems/goals/plans. Both should include variance tracking elements.	To individualise care for an individual patient without forgetting that the variance tracking has to be recorded to ensure these individual elements are 'met', or actioned accordingly if 'not met', whilst providing data for continuous improvements.
Make a check list of activities that will enable the collection and measurements of items that will want to be known clinically, administratively and managerially, to ensure they have each been included in the ICP.	This will ensure that data and information that is required at every level across the Trust is recorded once only and at the point of care of delivery. This avoids duplication of effort, separate activity and increased accuracy of data.

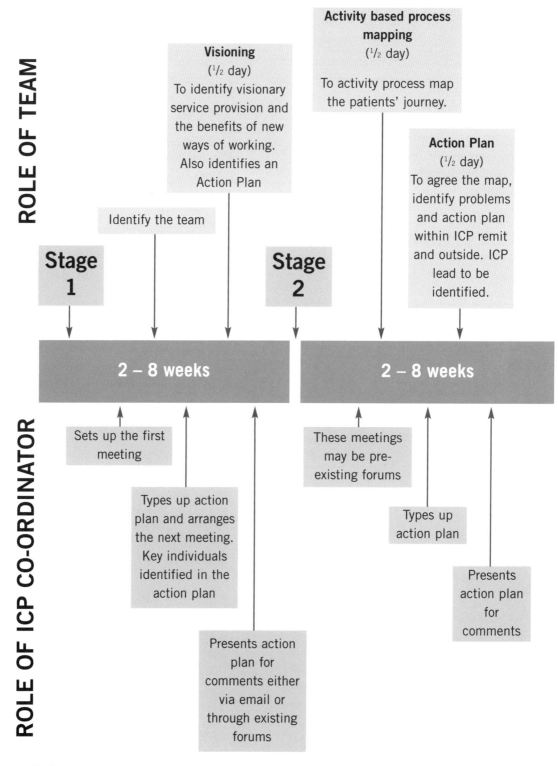

Visioning
(¹/₂ day)
To identify visionary service provision and the benefits of new ways of working. Also identifies an Action Plan

Activity based process mapping
(¹/₂ day)

To activity process map the patients' journey.

Action Plan
(¹/₂ day)
To agree the map, identify problems and action plan within ICP remit and outside. ICP lead to be identified.

Identify the team

ROLE OF TEAM

Stage 1

Stage 2

2 – 8 weeks

2 – 8 weeks

ROLE OF ICP CO-ORDINATOR

Sets up the first meeting

Types up action plan and arranges the next meeting. Key individuals identified in the action plan

Presents action plan for comments either via email or through existing forums

These meetings may be pre-existing forums

Types up action plan

Presents action plan for comments

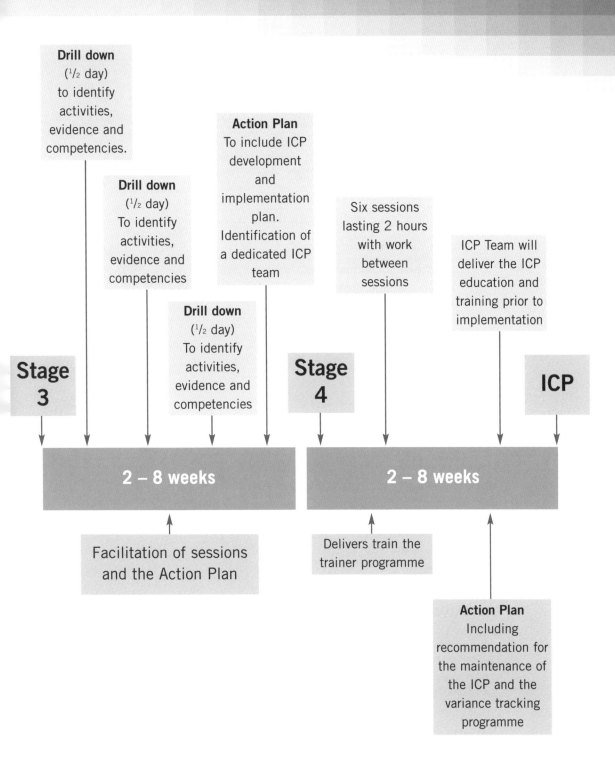

Drill down
(¹/₂ day)
to identify
activities,
evidence and
competencies.

Drill down
(¹/₂ day)
To identify
activities,
evidence and
competencies

Action Plan
To include ICP
development
and
implementation
plan.
Identification of
a dedicated ICP
team

Six sessions
lasting 2 hours
with work
between
sessions

ICP Team will
deliver the ICP
education and
training prior to
implementation

Drill down
(¹/₂ day)
To identify
activities,
evidence and
competencies

Stage 3

Stage 4

ICP

2 – 8 weeks

2 – 8 weeks

Facilitation of sessions
and the Action Plan

Delivers train the
trainer programme

Action Plan
Including
recommendation for
the maintenance of
the ICP and the
variance tracking
programme

Appendix 4 The Venture 'Good Integrated Care Pathway Template' Matrix©

Using the matrix below, appraise the ICP by ticking in the right-hand columns. If you can answer yes to a statement, tick the 'yes' column, if you can answer a definite 'no' or do not know, put a tick in the appropriate column. Count up what percentage of the statements for your ICP where you answered the statement with a 'yes'.

This matrix has been reproduced with the permission of Venture and Training Consultancy Ltd, Manor Farm Barns, Selsey Road, Donnington, Chichester, West Sussex PO20 7PL www.venturetc.com with thanks to Jenny Grey

Statement	Yes	No	Partly / Don't know
Consensus agreement was achieved for the layout of the ICP by all disciplines/members of the ICP project team			
The ICP was drafted with support of senior management			
The ICP puts the patient firmly at the centre of all activities			
All the relevant local and national guidelines/ protocols etc for the area of activity have been incorporated			
Sections or activities within the ICP that can be recorded/tracked by patients/carers and/or that involve patients in the agreement of their individual plans of care have been included			
There is room within the ICP for the recording of additional activities to individualise care for an individual patient			
Risks have been identified and risk assessment tools are embedded in the ICP			
All issues related to access and boundaries to seamless delivery of care (e.g. criteria for referral and discharge, pre-referral/pre-discharge/transfer actions, internal and external communications) have been included in the ICP			
All activities that will enable measurements of the impact of the ICP and production of follow up data to compare with any baseline audit data, have been included (refer to MinP)			
The ICP has a unique patient identifier on every page			

	Yes	No	Partly / Don't know
The ICP has a version control (number and date of issue) on every page			
The ICP has a recognisable look, so that all staff can recognise it as an ICP quickly and easily			
The title of the ICP is shown clearly on the front and then on every page			
The ICP has inclusion/exclusion criteria set out clearly, stating when the ICP should be used			
The explanation of how to use the ICP includes how (and where) to record variances when they occur			
The ICP has contact details for who to call if there are any queries regarding the ICP document			
The ICP has sample signatures and initials section at the front			
The ICP has activities set out in a clear manner			
The ICP has activity statements that are written using active rather than passive phrasing e.g. 'Secretary puts the Team Referral Form in the Consultant's tray' rather than 'Team Referral Form is put in the Consultant's tray', so that users can initial the activity as met or unmet			
It is clear for each activity 'who, what, when, where and why' (see Venture Guide to ICP Activity Writing)			
The activities describe the clinical and non clinical steps as they are; no folklore!			
Qualified terms are used to avoid ambiguity e.g 'Team Referral Form' rather than 'referral form'			
Synonyms are avoided e.g. referral form, form			
Abbreviations and jargon, when used, have been included e.g. 'Secretary puts the Team Referral Form in the Consultant's tray on the same day as it is received'			
Wherever appropriate an outcome has been included			
All activities set out a goal/success criteria that is objective and SMART i.e.Specific, Measurable, Achieved, Realistic, Timed			
Any evidence-based best practice has been referenced and recorded in a central, accessible database.			
Each activity in the ICP has an associated record for whether it was met/not met			
Each activity in the ICP has an associated section where the date and time of the activity can be recorded			
Each activity in the ICP has an associated section where the variance can be recorded			

	Yes	No	Partly / Don't know
The variance recording section enables the cause of the variance to be recorded			
The variance recording section enables the action taken as a result of the variance to be recorded			
The met/not met sections enable the initial of the person carrying out that element to be recorded			
The variances tracked when each activity is 'not met' provide a 'window of opportunity' to indicate that things have been missed or changed for a particular patient i.e. ensure that the ICP will act as an early warning signal and highlight trends that may lead to adverse incidents			
A section for recording individual patient 'problems/ goals/plan/notes' has been incorporated, with variance tracking of the 'problem/goal/plan' elements (or similar format)			
All activities covering the completion, sending, receiving, booking etc of all tests, charts, assessments, diagrams, letters, forms, information leaflets, satisfaction questionnaires, risk assessment tools, scales for measurement of clinical effectiveness, care planning etc have been included in the ICP			
The ICP pages are not over-crowded			
The ICP is written in a font size that is easy to read			
The ICP has a freehand recording section that can be used by everyone using the ICP			
The ICP is pleasing to the eye			
The ICP encourages staff to like and use it			
The ICP can be used to share information e.g. with patients/clients, carers, managers, referrers, commissioners, within the bounds of confidentiality			
The ICP can be used for induction, training and supervision of staff			
The ICP can be shared with information Management and Technology colleagues to assist the move to electronic ICPs underpinning the Electronic Patient Record			
The ICP is intuitive to use; is easy to follow and easy to record in, even if you have never seen it before			
Totals	Yes	No	Partly / Don't Know

Appendix 5 ICP Impact Plan and Evaluation

ICP Title: _____

Contact Name for this Plan: _____

Date Identified	Area to be measured/Potential Benefit	Standard to be achieved or success criteria	Method of Evaluation		Action required to realise benefits	Date Evaluated	Impact/ changes and improvements made to practice and outcome
			Baseline	Follow Up			
		Set the target to be achieved that is realistic and ambitious i.e. a realistic target that will stretch the team Express the target as a value, not as an improvement e.g. % of patients who follow an agreed protocol. How will you know you've reached your objective? Like your objectives the success criteria will be SMART	What data? How will it be gathered? Who will collect and analyse it?	What data? How will it be gathered? Who will collect and analyse it?	This will come from your Action and Milestones Gantt Chart		

Appendix 6 Glossary

Term	Acronym	Definition
Activity		i. Any specific deed, action or task. ii. All work done by a unit. Should be managed as units of time (eg bed days) or some other measure that takes account of *casemix* (see below).
Activity based process map		a plan that records each action using a noun and verb. It focuses on the patient experience.
Aim		A goal, purpose or direction.
Bottleneck		Part of the system where patient flow is obstructed, causing waits and delays. Bottlenecks are caused by inefficiencies in the system; ultimate limits in availability of key resources are *constraints* (see below).
Casemix		The acknowledgement that not all patients / procedures are equal in terms of resource requirements.
Caseweights		A way of measuring *casemix* (see above). Caseweights apply a value to each procedure or diagnosis type that takes account of resource utilisation.
Clinical Audit		The systematic and critical analysis of the quality of the clinical care.
Clinical Negligence Scheme For Trusts	CNST	
Commission for Healthcare Improvement	CHI	Commission established to accelerate improvement in patient care and healthcare value for money across England and Wales.

Term	Acronym	Definition
Constraint		The step or resource in a process that ultimately limits the volume going through the process. The constraint should be significant and high cost (see Bottleneck above).
Demand		All referrals from all sources into a service; demand should be measured in units of time or some other way of incorporating casemix, not simply patient numbers.
Framework		A structured plan or the basis of a project.
Functional process map		A plan which records the main stages but does not give every action in the process. It focuses on the service not the patient.
ICP Programme		The overall plan/schedule for the development and implementation of ICPs across the health and social care community. The ICP Programme will be on-going.
ICP Project		The plan for the development and implementation of an individual ICP across the health and/or social care community. The ICP Project will have a start and finish and will be part of the ICP Programme.
ICP Toolkit		A document that directs the user to develop and implement an ICP in a corporate manner. This corporate approach will allow the sharing of work across organisational boundaries.
ICP Variance		A deviation from an activity set out in an ICP.

Appendix 7 Useful Resources

Websites

Clinical Governance Support Team
www.cgsupport.nhs.uk

Commission for Health Improvement (2003)
www.chi.nhs.uk

http://www.design-council.org.uk/govtdesigntoolkit/tools/dev_swot.html

European Pathways Association
www.e-p-a.org

Institute for Healthcare Improvement
www.ihi.org

International journal of integrated care.
www.ijic.org/index.html

Journal of Integrated Care Pathways
www.rsmpress.co.uk/jicp.htm

National Electronic Library for Health Care Pathways Gateway
www.nelh.nhs.uk/carepathways

NICE. Principles for Best Practice in Clinical Audit:
http://www.nelh.nhs.uk/nice_bpca.asp

Protocol Based Care: *Underpinning Improvement*
www.nelh.nhs.uk/carepathways/cdrom

Primary care clinical Practice Guidelines
http://medicine.ucsf.edu/resources/guidelines

Protocol Based Care:
http://www.modernnhs.nhs.uk/scripts/default.asp?site_id=10&id=9061

Smart groups – ICPs
www.smartgroups.com/groups/clinicalpathways

The National Clinical Audit support programme
www.nhsia.nhs.uk/ncasp

Online Publications

ARIF: 'Are Integrated Care Pathways (ICPs) effective and cost effective, particularly in terms of getting research evidence into practice?'
http://www.bham.ac.uk/arif/pathway.htm

Barker, A. & Frosdick, P. (1999) *Integrated Pathways of Care The Pharmaceutical Journal* Vol 263 No 7075 p950-951 December 11, 1999
Articles:
http://www.pharmj.com/Editorial/19991211/articles/pathways_care.html

Davis, M. (2004) Way to Go. Health Service Journal 13th May 2004
www.hsj.co.uk

National Prescribing Centre. *Implementing NICE Guidance: A practical handbook for professionals.* July 2001:
http://nww.npc.ppa.nhs.uk/publications/nice/nice.htm

Tunnicliffe, C.A. *Guidelines for the Development of Integrated Care Pathways Part 1 Guidance Framework and Audit Criteria.* (Version 1 June 2002).
Unpublished work.
Tunnicliffe, C.A. *Guidelines for the Development of Integrated Care Pathways Part 2 Audit Document.* (Version 1 June 2002). Unpublished work. Pembs & Derwen Intranet Site:
http://nww.pdt-tr.wales.nhs.uk/pdttr/index.htm

The National Assembly for Wales Value for Money Unit: 'Care Pathways'.
http://howis.wales.nhs.uk/doclib/preface_e.htm

References and Bibliography

Abu Own, A., Sachs, R., Louden, C., Linnard, D. and Buckland, J. (1999) Vascular Surgical Society of Great Britain and Ireland: integrated care pathways for vascular surgery *British Journal of Surgery* 86 (5): 703

Arragon, D., Burton, V., Byers, J.F. and Cohen, M. (2002) The effect of a critical pathway on patients' outcomes after carotid endarterectomy. *American Journal of Critical Care* May 11 (3): 250-158

Atwal, A. and Caldwell, K. (2002) Do multidisciplinary care pathways improve interprofessional collaboration: *Scandinavian Journal of Caring Sciences* Vol 16 P4

Bergman, B. and Klefsjo, B. (1994) *Quality from Customer Needs to Customer Satisfaction.* McGraw Hill. London.

Crosby, Philip B. (1996) *Quality is Still Free:* Making Quality Certain in Uncertain Times. McGraw Hill, New York

Currie L, Harvey G (1998) Care pathways development and implementation. *Nursing Standard* 12, 30, 35-38

Dykes, P.C. (1998) *Psychiatric Clinical Pathways: An Interdisciplinary Approach* Connecticut: Aspen Publishers Inc.

De Luc, K., Kitchiner, D., Layton, A., Morris, E., Murray, Y. and Overill, S. (2001) *Developing Care Pathways the Handbook.* Oxon: Radcliffe Medical Press Ltd

De Luc, K., Kitchiner, D., Layton, A., Morris, E., Murray, Y. and Overill, S. (2001) *Developing Care Pathways the Tool Kit.* Oxon: Radcliffe Medical Press Ltd

De Luc, K. & Todd, J. (2003) *e-Pathways computers and the patient's journey.* Radcliffe, Medical Press Ltd.

De Luc, K. (2002) *Developing Care Pathways: The Handbook* National Pathways Association Radcliffe Medical Press

Edwards, A. & Elwyn, G. (Eds) (2001) *Evidence Based Patient Choice: Inevitable or Impossible* Oxford University Press

Gray, J. (2004) The dawning of a new era *Journal of Integrated Care Pathways* (2004) 8, 1-2

Guezo, J. (2003) Total Abdominal Hysterectomy: Development of a patient centred care pathway *Nursing Standard* P 38-42 Vol 18 No 3

Hornby, S. *Collaborative Care Interprofessional, Interagency and Interpersonal* Oxford Blackwell Scientific Publications 1993

Johnson, S. (1997) *Pathways of Care* Blackwell Science

Johnson, S. (2001) *Journal of Integrated Care Pathways.* 5(1), April 2001. West Sussex: The Royal Society of Medicine Press Ltd

Johnson, S. (2001) *Journal of Integrated Care Pathways.* 7(2), August 2003. West Sussex: The Royal Society of Medicine Press Ltd

Jones, T. (2002) cited in Middleton, S. & Roberts, A. (Eds), *Integrated Care Pathways: A practical approach to implementation* Butterworth Heinemann. Oxford

Jones, T., De Luc, K. and Coyne, H. (1999) *Managing Care Pathways the Quality and Resources of Hospital Care.* London: The Certified Accountants Educational Trust (CAET).

Jones, T., Hardwick, A. and Curruthers, I. (2000) *New Commissioning applying Integrated Care Pathways.* London: The Certified Accountants Educational Trust (CAET).

Jones, T., and Coyne, H. (2001) *Modernisation and Care Pathways ICP Symposium.* London: The Certified Accountants Educational Trust (CAET)

Juran (1992) *Juran on Quality by Design* McGraw-Hill, New York

Mackay, L., Soothail, K. & Webb, C (1995) cited in Soothill, K., Mackay, L. & Webb, C. (Eds) *Interprofessional Relations in Healthcare* Edward Arnold. London

Middleton, S., Barnett, J. and Reeves, D. (2001) *What is an Integrated Care Pathway?* 3(3), February 2001. Hayward Medical Communications.

Middleton, S. & Roberts, A. (2003) *Integrated Care Pathways: A Practical Approach to Implementation.* Butterworth, Heinemann.

Naidoo, M. and Bullock, R. (2001) *An Integrated Care Pathway for Dementia Best Practice for Dementia Care.* Swindon: Harcourt Health Communications

National Assembly of Wales (1998) *Better Health, Better Wales* NHS Cymru

National Assembly of Wales (2001) *Improving Health in Wales: A Plan for the NHS and its Partners* NHS Cymru

NHS Cymru Wales (September 1999). *An Introduction to Clinical Pathways; putting patients first.* The National Assembly for Wales.

Nursing Times (2003). *Protocol Based Care.* London: Emap Healthcare Ltd

Parsley, K. & Corrigan, P. (1999) *Quality Improvement in Healthcare: Putting Evidence into Practice* 2nd Edition Stanley Thornes

Roberts, A. and Middleton, S. (2000) *Integrated Care Pathways A practical approach to Implementation.* Oxford: Butterworth

Sale, D. (1997) *Quality Assurance A Pathway to Excellence* McMillan Press

Sulch, D, Kalra, L. (2000) *Integrated Care Pathways in Stroke Management* Age Ageing July 29 (4): 349-52

Thompson, D. and Wright, K. (2003). *Developing a Unified Patient Record a practical guide.* Oxon: Radcliffe Medical Press

Walsh, M. (1997) *Models and Critical Pathways in Clinical Nursing* Baillieree Tindall

Welsh Assembly Government (2005) *Designed for Life: Creating World Class Health and Social Care for Wales in the 21st Century*

White, T. *Are you falling down in the prevention of falls? Changing the delivery of care through the development and implementation of a multidisciplinary assessment tool and care pathways.*
Journal of Integrated Care Pathways (2004) 8, 19-26